YOUR KNOWLEDGE HAS VALUE

AF136907

- We will publish your bachelor's and master's thesis, essays and papers

- Your own eBook and book - sold worldwide in all relevant shops

- Earn money with each sale

Upload your text at www.GRIN.com and publish for free

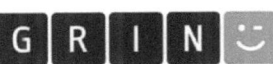

Bibliographic information published by the German National Library:

The German National Library lists this publication in the National Bibliography; detailed bibliographic data are available on the Internet at http://dnb.dnb.de .

Imprint:

Copyright © 2018 GRIN Verlag
Print and binding: Books on Demand GmbH, Norderstedt Germany
ISBN: 9783346218155

This book at GRIN:

https://www.grin.com/document/594788

Kim Stewart

Medical Marijuana as Alternative to Opiates. Does it Reduce Pain and Improve the Quality of Living?

GRIN Verlag

GRIN - Your knowledge has value

Since its foundation in 1998, GRIN has specialized in publishing academic texts by students, college teachers and other academics as e-book and printed book. The website www.grin.com is an ideal platform for presenting term papers, final papers, scientific essays, dissertations and specialist books.

Visit us on the internet:

http://www.grin.com/

http://www.facebook.com/grincom

http://www.twitter.com/grin_com

Literature Review on the Effect of using Cannabis with or instead of Opioids on the Quality of

Life in Patients Suffering with Chronic Pain

Kim E. Stewart

University of Central Florida

EFFECT OF CANNABIS ON PAIN AND QUALITY OF LIFE

Abstract

Deaths due to opioid overdose continues to rise to the point that opioid use is now considered an epidemic. Since opioids are the common prescribed drug to treat chronic pain, there is a need to consider safer alternate treatments. This integrated literature review was conducted to examine if cannabis can effectively treat pain, improve quality of life, and reduce the need for opioids to manage chronic pain. Nine studies were included in this review. All nine studies reported the effectiveness of cannabis in either pain management, decreased opioid use and/or improved quality of life. Because consideration of the medicinal uses of cannabis is new, eight of the nine studies included less than a one year follow up. However, the results of the studies reveal that cannabis should be considered for more than recreational uses and that its medicinal uses date back for thousands of years. To fully understand all the benefits and potential side effects surrounding cannabis, further research is needed. For further research to be conclusive, it is necessary for regulatory barriers and campaigns to reduce stigmas surrounding cannabis to be at the forefront. Deaths related to opioid overdose is in upward of 4 million people worldwide, including prescribed and illegal use compared to the absence of deaths related to cannabis overdose, a powerful indicator that cannabis may be the solution to help the millions of persons who suffer from chronic pain.

Keywords: cannabis, medical marijuana, quality of life, pain management, chronic pain, sleep quality, opioid reduction

2

Table of Contents

The Effect of using Cannabis with or instead of Opioids on the Quality of Life in Patients Suffering with Chronic Pain

The Institute of Medicine (n.d.) reports that chronic pain affects more than 100 million Americans and cost between $560-$635 billion dollars annually. Presently, opioids are the most common treatment for chronic pain suffers. The use and overuse of opioids has created an official "war on opioids" following an increasing number of opioid related deaths and dependence. It is critical that the medical community join the efforts to reduce opioid dependence and consider alternate measures to manage chronic pain. The Institute of Medicine (n.d.) promotes a comprehensive and interdisciplinary approach to the management of pain. For the past 4000 years, Cannabis has been utilized in society to create clothing, weapons and to treat a wide range of health-related disparities including chronic pain. Necessary research related to the efficacy and medicinal uses of Cannabis has been impeded by stigmas and regulatory barriers. Current yet limited research concludes that cannabis is an effective treatment for the management of chronic pain. Additionally, patients using cannabis to treat pain report an enhanced quality of life and reduction of opioid use.

Background and Significance

According to the Centers for Disease Control and Prevention (2016), there were more than 249 million opioid prescriptions written for the management of chronic pain in the United States. Although opioids have long been considered the most effective treatment for the management of pain, the consequences to their use and overuse has recently been brought to the attention of healthcare providers as well as government agencies. The U.S. Department of Health and Human Services estimates that 11.5 million people have misused prescription opioids and that 2.1 million people are diagnosed with an opioid use disorder. Prolonged opioid use not only places the chronic pain patient at risk of addiction but also at risk for loss of employability often resulting in financial burden. Several other risk factors are associated with prolonged opioid use including bowel dysfunction, reduced cognition and increased hospital stays but the greatest concern is in the year 2016 more than 42,000 people died from overdosing on opioids (U.S. Department of Health and Human Services, 2017). According to Rudd, Aleshire, Zibbell & Gladden (2016), in the year 2014, 1.5 times more deaths were attributed to opioid overdose than to motor vehicle accidents. The U.S. Department of Health and Human Services (2017) estimates that opioid use and misuse creates a 504-billion-dollar economic cost on an annual basis. The opioid epidemic currently litters both local and national news daily.

Simultaneous to the opioid epidemic, the legalization and use of cannabis has splashed headline news. According to Robinson, Berke & Gould (2018) medical marijuana is legal in 30 states including the District of Columbia and recreational marijuana is legal in nine of those states. Although cannabis has a wide range of uses, according to Bushak, (2016) cannabis and its three species and several sub species has been used in medicine for thousands of years. Cannabis use dates to ancient China when it was used to make tea used to treat health disparities such as gout, rheumatism, and malaria. Between 2000-1400 B.C. India commonly used marijuana to treat digestive problems, increase appetite and provide alertness to the mind (Bushak, 2016). In the early 1900's marijuana was introduced into the U.S. by Mexican immigrants and was considered a recreational drug for low class people. In 1970, Marijuana became categorized as a Schedule I drug meaning that there is no suggested medical use and it has a high risk of addiction and death. Between the 1960's and 1970's marijuana became affiliated with the hippie movement and considered a mind altering psychedelic drug. Marijuana quickly became one of the drugs in which the task force for drug prevention and the Drug Enforcement Agency targeted for extinction and for which persons were criminalized for possession. A lot has changed since the 1970's, the

5

National Academics of Sciences Engineering Medicine (2017) pubically released a presentation on the current state of evidence and recommendations for research regarding the benefits of cannabis and cannabinoids. The esteemed committee concluded there are several health-related benefits to cannabinoids including the management of nausea and vomiting, reduction of pain in chronic pain patients and the reduction of spasticity in persons with multiple sclerosis. In comparison to the daily 116 deaths related to opioid overdose and the annual 42,000 deaths per year related to opioid overdose, the Drug Enforcement Administration (n.d.) reports the death toll related to cannabis overdose to total zero, in its entire documented history.

Current research falls short in illustrating conclusive evidence relating to the use of cannabinoids and its effect on pain management and quality of life. There is a need for research that institutes standard measures and methodologies while addressing the long-term effects of cannabis for the management of chronic pain. Some possible barriers to research include the regulatory barriers that surround Medical Marijuana as it remains a Schedule I substance which further complicates availability in obtaining different strains of cannabis and studying them for efficacy. Without full access to a variety cannabis strains, research and conclusive evidence relating to short and long-term health related outcomes are difficult to conclude. Additionally, stigmas surrounding medical marijuana may have an impact on the acceptability when considering it for positive medical outcomes. Medical professionals demand increased evidence based facts regarding the prescriptive qualities and efficacy of prescribing cannabis as an adjunct or in place of opioid treatment for chronic pain. Persons who suffer with chronic pain management deserve effective treatment with lowered risk of harm.

The purpose of this review is to determine if the use of cannabis can improve the quality of life in persons suffering from chronic pain. For the purpose of this review, quality of life is defined by the factors of reduced pain, less dependence on opioids, sleep quality and social functioning.

6

Method

A search strategy was performed to identify English written works published between 1999-2018. The following databases were utilized in the search strategy: CINAHL-Plus with Full Text, HealthWatch, MEDLINE, Cochrane Database of Systematic Reviews and PsycINFO. The search included the following key words; Medical Marijuana, Dronabinol, Cannabidiol, Cannabinoids, Delta 9, Tetracannabinol, cannabinoid, opioid, opiates, narcotics, chronic pain, persistent pain, long term pain, quality of life, compare and evaluation. The search excluded studies utilizing animal subjects. Articles were included and further reviewed if they included individual case studies although low level of evidence. Further reviews were conducted when articles included both medical marijuana or alternative term, opioid usage, quality of life and reduction in opioid usage. Articles were excluded when they related to single subject, either marijuana or opioid use, historical use of marijuana, laws that govern marijuana use, series of incomplete studies, studies concerning drug abuse and informational self-reports. Criteria provided by Ebell, Siwek, Weiss, Woolf, Susman, Ewigman & Bowman (2004) was utilized to determine study quality and appropriate levels of evidence.

Search Results

Searches of the electronic databases resulted in forty-nine articles. Of those, thirty-three articles were eliminated due to a variety of factors. The majority of elimination factors included articles whose primary focus on historical marijuana use and laws that govern medical marijuana. Additionally, a number of articles were eliminated due to primarily focused on opioid use and abuse. Two articles were eliminated due to being part of an incomplete series and two articles were individual self-reports of cannabis use. Two articles were included in the review, although are case reports with low levels of evidence, both are relevant to the topic of medical marijuana

7

use along with opioid use and quality of life and offer specific benefits of cannabis use. According to Ebell et al. (2004), two studies offer Level 1 quality and Level A strength with consistent results (Narang et al., 2008 and Johnson et al., 2010), with the remaining studies falling within the Level 2 quality and Level B strength. In consideration of the newness on the use of medical marijuana for pain management, the two case study reports are included in this review and offer outstanding personalized patient experiences. Appendix A summarizes the nine articles including their focus, design method, sample/setting, major variables studied, intervention, measurement, data analysis and findings and appraisal.

Major themes considered as part of this integrated literature review include the effects of including cannabis for chronic pain on: quality of life, pain management, decreased opioid use, sleep quality and social functioning.

Integrated Findings

The nine studies included 4155 participants in total. All the studies included participants with previous experience using cannabis, either medicinally or recreationally. All the studies utilized cannabis or a derivative to address pain, opioid use reduction or to enhance quality of life. All nine studies utilized varied forms of cannabis administration. Five studies utilized smoked cannabis as the route of administration including; (Haroutounion et al., 2016; Lynch, P., 2012; Johnson et al., 2010; Reynolds et al., 2013; and Ware et al., 2016). Three studies included participants enrolled in a Medical Cannabis Program (MCP) that offered different forms of cannabis via smokable or edible depending on participant preference, including; (Boehnke et al., 2016; Reiman, Welty, & Solomon, 2017; & Vigil et al., 2017). One study utilized cannabis strictly in the form of capsules in 10mg or 20mg strength, Narang et al., (2008). All the studies included participants suffering with some form of chronic pain, however one study did not report the effects of the utilization of cannabis on chronic pain and focused mainly on the reduction of opioid usage (Boehnke et al., 2016).

Themes

Three themes emerged from this integrated literature review: The effect of cannabis on pain management, the reduction of opioid use when adding cannabis to a pain medication regime and the effect on quality of life when using cannabis in addition to or instead of opioids for pain management. According to Niv & Kreitler, (2001) Pain is responsible for affecting most domains of quality of life including physical and emotional functioning.

Pain Management

Eight of nine studies including 3781 participants reported the effect of cannabis on the management of chronic pain. All eight studies reported results indicating pain reduction when cannabis was added to their pain management plan. Two studies utilized the Brief Pain Inventory Short Form a nine-question survey utilizing a (0 least pain -10 most pain) Likert Scale to indicate the degree in which pain effects the participants life as well as rating the degree of pain itself; (Haroutounion et al., 2016; and Narong et al., 2008) with significant pain reduction in their respective 200 participants, with significance ranging from p<0.001 to p<0.01. Two studies utilized a Numeric Rating Scale reporting significant pain improvement in their 243 participants (Johnson et al., 2010; and Vigil et al., 2017) The Vigil et al., (2017) reported significant mean pain reduction from baseline to post study of 3.4 points p<0.001. Haroutouunion et al., (2016) utilized both the BPI and the S-TOPS tools for measurements of pain baseline and at study completion. The remaining studies used a variety of tools to determine pain levels pre- and post-study. Two studies were case studies although with lower levels of evidence report one subject (Reynold, D.

& Osborn, H., 2013) and three subjects (Lynch, P., 2012) success in reducing pain levels when introducing cannabis to the participants medication regime. In the Lynch, P. (2012) study, two of three participants reported life changing pain relief and one participant, although did not report pain relief was able to discontinue the use of opioids altogether, presuming that he too experienced pain relief. The Reynold, D. & Osborn, H. (2013) study was a single participant study where the participant reported life altering benefits after adding cannabis to his pain management regime and even able to tolerate hugging loved ones, shaving and going out in the colder weather after facial skin cancer surgery's stole his abilities to do so for years prior to the study participation. The Narang et al., (2008) study, a randomized single-dose double-blinded placebo controlled crossover trial reported that there was no statistical difference in pain relief between the low dose dronabinol (a cannabinoid strain)10mg and the high dose dronabinol 20mg with regards to pain relief, indicating that higher doses of cannabis did not produce greater pain relief, however did produce higher pain relief over the placebo dronabinol vs placebo average pain intensity $p<0.001$).

The results of these eight studies reports that patients who suffer with chronic pain find greater pain relief when adding cannabis to their pain management regime over using opioids alone to manage their symptoms.

Opioid Reduction

Five of the nine studies including 3327 participants reported levels of opioid reduction when adding cannabis to their pain management regime. According to the U.S. Department of Health and Human Services (2017) more than 42,000 people died from overdosing on opioid medications and with prolonged use can also lead to increase hospital stays, bowel dysfunction and reduced cognition. To improve the quality of life in persons suffering with chronic pain who are prescribed opioids for pain management, the consideration of adding cannabis to their pain

10

management is considered. Three of the five studies included participants enrolled in a Medical Cannabis Program (MCP) where distribution of the prescribed amounts of cannabis were managed, (Boehnke et al., 2016; Reiman et al., 2017; and Vigil et al., 2017). The Boehnke et al., (2016) study reported participants experienced a 45% decrease in opioid use after adding cannabis to their medication regime 119/184 (65%) used opioids before cannabis and 33/184 (18%) after cannabis. Perhaps the most robust results were reported in the Vigil et al. (2017) study where persons who ceased opioid post cannabis intervention using a means comparison 3.4% vs MCP 40.5% = p<0.001 and those who reduced prescribed daily opioid dosage means comparison 44.8% vs 83.8% MCP =p 0.001 with conclusions including that medical cannabis reduced opioid use in 80% of MCP participants and ceased opioid use in 40% of participants. The Reiman et al., (2017) study utilized a patient self-report Likert scale to determine levels of agreement regarding cannabis use and opioid use. The Reiman et al., (2017) study reported that 97% of participants strongly agreed/agreed that they could decrease opiate dosage when initiating cannabis for pain management. The Haroutounion et al., (2016) and Lynch, P. (2012) studies did not include participants enrolled in an MCP. The Haroutounion et al., (2016) study reported that 32 of the 73 participants discontinued opioid use (41 vs 73, p<0.001) representing a 44% reduction and the medium opioid dose decreased from 60mg (95% CI, 45.0-90.0) to 45mg (95% CI, 30.0-90.0) daily however did not reach significance (p=0.19 using the Means Whitney test). The Lynch, P., (2012) study, a case study with three participants including the following opioid reduction and cessation, see figure 1:

figure 1

Participant	Daily Opioid Dosage Prior to Cannabis	Daily Opioid Dosage After Cannabis
Patient One (Chronic Multiple Sclerosis)	Morphine 75mg Daily	Morphine 45mg daily (after 6 months) (-35mg daily)
Patient Two (HIV Positive Peripheral Neuropathy)	Morphine 300mg Long Acting Daily	Morphine 180mg after 4 months and after 9 months Morphine discontinued (-110mg then -300mg daily)
Patient Three (Low Back and Leg Pain due to fall onto a metal tank)	Morphine 150mg Long Acting Daily	Morphine 90mg daily after 2 weeks and after 4 weeks Morphine 60mg daily. (-60mg then -90mg daily)

*Lynch, P. (2012) Case Study Result

The results of these five studies illustrate that chronic pain patients can reduce and cease the use of opioid medications when adding cannabis to their pain management regime. The cessation and reduction of the use of opioids benefits the patient by reducing the risks of death related to overdose, increased hospitalizations, bowel dysfunction, cognitive function and overall functioning and quality of life.

Quality of Life (sleep and social functioning)

Quality of life (QOL) is defined as "the person's evaluation of his or her well-being and functioning in different life domains, Niv & Kreitler, (2001)". QOL is a subjective state of being and may change over the duration and intensity of any disease process. QOL includes sleep quality as well as social functioning, both the focus of this review.

Six of the nine studies including 716 participants reported results on QOL related to adding cannabis to medication regime for chronic pain management. Two of the six studies (Narang et al., 2008; and Ware et al., 2015) reported QOL outcomes utilizing the same tool of measurement, the RAND SF-36 which is a short form health survey that can measure quality of life. Higher RAND scores represent a higher quality of life. The Narang et al., (2008) also utilized the MOS Sleep Scale, a 12-item self-reporting measure to determine quality of sleep in patients with chronic pain. The results of the SF-36 were similar between the two studies. The Narang et al. (2008)

12

study reports RAND scores showing improvement at the end of the study with respect to Social Functioning p<0.01 and MOS Sleep Scale Scores showing a decrease in sleep disturbance after treatment p<0.01 with an increase in sleep adequacy p<0.05. The Ware et al., (2015) study reported significant improvements in QOL ccmparing baseline, 6 month and 12 months post treatment (6 month: 2.36 points greater improvement 95% CI=.84-3.98 and at 12 months: 1.62 points 95% CI=010-3.14). Two studies utilized a patient self-report questionnaire, (Boehnke et al.; 2016) and Vigil et al., 2017). The Boehnke et al (2016) study reports that side effects of everyday functioning decreased after the initiation of cannabis (6.51 vs 2.79 p<0.001) and the Vigil et al., (2017) reports that; 65% of participants showed a good or great benefit to the addition of medical cannabis about their QOL, 52% of participants reported good or great benefit to their social life, 67% to their activity levels and 41% reported gcod or great benefit to their concentration levels. The two-remaining study's, Lynch, P., (2012) and Reynolds D. & Osborn, H., (2013), case studies, reported individual QOL improvements after the initiation of medical cannabis including; sleep, ability to continue working, being able to go outside after 4 years, being able to shave and being able to tolerate hugs from loved ones.

The results of these six studies reveal that there is benefit to adding medical cannabis to chronic pain patients including improved QOL/Social Functioning and Sleep Quality. Improvements in QOL for persons suffering with chronic pain is substantial to the success of long term management of health-related disparities. Cannabis may allow patients to regain enjoyment of social and recreational activities which lead to optimal functioning and greater patient satisfaction during the management of chronic pain events and disparities.

Limitations of Evidence

Only one study compared the effects of varied cannabis milligrams to placebo (Narang et al., 2008). One study compared two different strains of cannabis (Johnson et al., 2010). Only two studies utilized the same measurement tool, the Brief Pain Inventory (Haroutounion et al., 2016; and Narang et al., 2008). Two studies were approved by the institutional review board (Reinman et al., 2017; and Vigil et al., 2017). The Ware et al, (2015) study included a one year follow up, and the remaining 8 studies were of shorter duration. The Reiman et al., (2017) study was adequate in size with 2897 participants, however may have been biased due to offering a chance to win a gift for participation. The Narang et al., (2008) study contained the highest level of evidence and the highest quality of evidence using a randomized single-dose double-blinded placebo controlled crossover trial in two phases. No studies identified participants whom had no experience with cannabis, medicinally or recreationally.

Recommendations

Further research is necessary to address the long-term effects and all the medicinal uses for cannabis. Future research should not be hindered by regulatory barriers therefore legislative efforts to remove medical marijuana from its schedule II status should be supported by health-care professionals. For medical cannabis to be accepted for its medicinal purposes, public campaigns and focused education to the medical community is necessary to remove the stigma surrounding its use. Future researchers should adapt a preferred method of measurement to compare multiple study results. Future research should also consider studies that compare a variety of cannabis strands and dosage amounts which will offer prescribers more confidence when considering cannabis for medicinal use. Anecdotical evidence and limited research findings support the use of medicinal cannabis as an approach to manage pain, improve quality of life, and help the war on

14

opioid dependence and overdose therefore it is essential that there is adequate funding for necessary research to propel it's use to its fullest potential.

Conclusion

Although this review was limited to small number of studies, they did reveal conclusive and not generalizable evidence that cannabis can provide pain relief, reduce opioid use, and improve quality of life. In consideration that the number of people who suffer from chronic pain continues to rise, primary medical treatment for chronic pain is opioids and the fact that opioids can reduce quality of life and lead to dependence an unintentional overdose, it is essential that all alternate treatments for chronic pain are considered. While these studies report that cannabis can provide safe pain relief and improve quality of life its current regulatory barriers and stigma has impeded the necessary research which would allow researchers to examine the long-term safety and any side effects that need to be identified to insure public safety prior to public use.

References

Boehnke, K., Litinas, E. & Clauw, D. (2016). Medical cannabis use is associated with decreased opiate medication use in retrospective cross-sectional survey of patients with chronic pain. *The Journal of Pain 17(6).*

Bushak, L. (2016). A brief history of medical cannabis: From ancient anesthesia to the modern Dispensary. *The Grapevine.* Retrieved from http://www.medicaldaily.com/brief-history- medical-cannabis-ancient-anesthesia-modern-dispensary-370344

Centers for Disease Control and Prevention (CDC) (2016). CDC guideline for prescribing opioids for chronic pain. Retrieved from: https://www.cdc.gov/drugoverdose/pdf/guidelines_at-a-glance-a.pdf

Centers for Disease Control and Prevention (CDC) (2017). Opioid Overdose. Retrieved from: https://www.cdc.gov/drugoverdose/

Drug Enforcement Agency (n.d.) Drug fact sheet. Marijuana. Retrieved from: https://www.dea.gov/druginfo/drug_data_sheets/Marijuana.pdf

Ebell, M., Siwek, J., Weiss, B, Woolf, S., Susman, J., Ewigman, B. & Bowman, M. (2004). Simplifying the language of evidence to improve patient care. American Family Physician (69)3. Pp 548-749. Retrieved from file:///C:/Users/kimsr_000/Downloads/Simplifying_the_language_of_ev%20(1).PDF

Frank, B., Serpell, M., Hughes, J. Matthews, J. & Kapur, D. (2007) Comparison of analgesic effects and patient tolerability of nabi8lone and dihydrocodeine for chronic neuropathic pain: randomized, crossover, double blind study. *BMJ Research.* Doi: 10.1136/bmj.39429.619653.80

Governing (2018) State marijuana laws in 2018 map. Retrieved from:

http://www.governing.com/gov-data/state-marijuana-laws-map-medical-recreational.html

Haroutounion, S., Ratz, Y., Ginosar, Y., Furmanov, K., Saifi, F, Meidan, R. & Davidson, E. (2016). The effect of medicinal cannabis on pain and quality-of-life outcomes in chronic pain. *Clinical Journal of Pain 32*(12). pp 1036-1043.

Hill, K., Palastro, M., Johnson, B., & Ditre, J. (2017). Cannabis and pain: A clinical review. Cannabis and Cannabinoid Research (2) 1. DOI: 10.1089/can.207 0017.

Institute of Medicine (n.d.) Institute of medicine: Relieving pain in America. Retrieved from: https://iprcc.nih.gov/sites/default/files/IOM_Pain_Report_508comp_0.pdf

Johnson, J., Burnell-Nugent, M, Lossignol, D, Ganae-Motan, E, Potts, R. & Fallon, M. (2010). Multicenter, double-blind, randomized, placebo-controlled, parallel-group study of the efficacy, safety, and tolerability of thc: cbd extract and thc extract in patients with intractable cancer related pain. *Journal of Pain and Symptom Management 39*(2). Doi: 10.1016/j.ipainsymman.2009.06.008

Kossen, J. (2016). *Is cannabis better for chronic pain than opiods?* Leafly. Retrieved from: https://www.leafly.com/news/health/cannabis-for-chronic-pain-vs-opioids

Lynch, P. (2012). Cannabis as an adjunct to or substitute for opiates in the treatment of chronic pain. *Journal of Psychoactive Drugs, 44*(2).

Mole, E. (2017). World health organization clashes with dea on marijuana compound cbd. Ars TECHNICA. Retrieved from: https://arstechnica.com/science/2017/12/who-report-data-on-marijuana-compound-does-not-justify-dea-scheduling/

Narang, S., Gibson, D., Wasan, A., Ross, E., Michna, E., Nedeljkovic, S.& Jamison, R. (2008). Efficacy of dronabinol as an adjuvant treatment for chronic pain patients on opioid therapy. *The Journal of Pain 5(3).* pp 254-264.

National Institute on Drug Abuse (NIDA) (2018). *Misuse of Prescription Drugs.* Retrieved from https://www.drugabuse.gov/publications/research-reports/misuse-prescription-drugs on

Niv, D. & Kreitler, S. (2001). Pain and quality of life. *Pain Practice (1)*2. Retrieved from: https://www.ncbi.nlm.nih.gov/pubmed/17129291

Randolph, J. (2009). A guide to writing the dissertation literature review. *Practical assessment, research & evaluation. (14)* 13. Retrieved from: http://pareonline.net/pdf/v14n13.pdf

Reiman, A., Welty, M. & Solomon, P. (2017). Cannabis a a substitute for opioid-based pain medication: Patient self-report. *Cannabis and Cannabinoid Research 2*(1).

Reynolds, D. & Osborn, H. (2013). The use of cannabinoids in chronic pain. *BMJ Case Report*. Doi: 10.1136/bcr-2013-010417.

Robinson, M., Berke, J. & Gould, S. (2018). *This map shows every state that has legalized Marijuana*. Business Insider. Retrieved from: http://www.businessinsider.com/legal-marijuana-states-2018-1

Rudd, R., Aleshire, N., Zibbell, J. & Gladden, M. (2016). Increases in drug and opioid overdose Deaths-united states, 2000-2014. *CDC Morbidity and Mortality Weekly Report*. Retrieved from https://www.cdc.gov/mmwr/preview/mmwrhtml/mm6450a3.htm?s_cid= mm6450a3_w

The National Academics of Sciences Engineering Medicine (2017). Health effects of cannabis and cannabinoids. Retrieved from:

http://nationalacademies.org/hmd/~/media/Files/Report%20Files/2017/Cannabis-Health-Effects/Cannabis-public-release-slides.pdf

Vigil, J., Stith, S., Adams, I. & Reeves, A. (2017). Associations between medical cannabis and prescription opiod use in chronic pain patients: A preliminary cohort study. *PLOS ONE 12(11)*. Doi: 106084/m9figshare.5671721

U.S. Department of Health and Human Services (2017). The u.s. opioid epidemic. Retrieved from https://www.hhs.gov/opioids/about-the-epidemic/

Ware, M., Wang, T., Shapiro, S. & Collet, J. (2015). Cannabis for the management of pain: Assessment of safety study. Journal of Pain 16(12). Pp 1233-1242.

EFFECT OF CANNABIS ON PAIN AND QUALITY OF LIFE

Appendix A

Evidence Evaluation Tables

Citation	Conceptual Framework	Design/Method	Sample/Setting	Major Variables Studied and Their Definitions	Measurement	Data Analysis	Findings	Appraisal: Worth to Practice
Boehnke, K., Litinas, E. & Clauw, D. (2016). Medical cannabis use is associated with decreased opiate medication use in retrospective cross-sectional survey of patients with chronic pain. *The Journal of Pain* 17(6).	N/A	Retrospective Cross-Sectional Survey (over 4 quarters)	N=185 Medical Cannabis Patients participating at the Michigan Medical Cannabis Dispensary between Nov, 2013 and February 2015	IV= Participants at the Ann Arbor, Michigan Medical Cannabis Dispensary DV: Changes in Opioid Use, Quality of Life, Medication classes used and Medication Side effects.	Survey Instrument: (46 questions) Changes in Opioid Use, Quality of Life, Medication Classes Used and Medication Side Effects Fibromyalgia Survey (0 to 31, 31 equals highest level of fibromyalgia pain)	Descriptive Statistics (fully completed questionnaires) Pearson Correlation Test T-Tests Analysis of Variance Tests	Mean number of medication classes decreased in all participants post cannabis use p<0.001 64% of participants showed a decrease in opioid use. 43% of participants showed improved quality of life. Decreased side effects of medication on everyday functioning p<0.001 Correlation between reduction of opioid use and decreased medication side effects significantly correlated: p=0.0002	**Limitations:** Study was exempted from institutional review board oversight Cross-Sectional Study Design limits inference of data become the outcomes of interest were measured with potentially unreliable recall data. No baseline data for Fibromyalgia Scores Unable to generalize findings due to only surveying population at medical cannabis dispensary. Opioid decrease may be a result of recent Newsline attention to opioid over use. Selection Bias **Strengths:** Significant decrease in side effects that effect daily functioning, decrease in total number of medications taken and improvements in quality of life.

EFFECT OF CANNABIS ON PAIN AND QUALITY OF LIFE

Citation	Conceptual Framework	Design/Method	Sample/Setting	Major Variables Studied and Their Definitions	Measurement	Data Analysis	Findings	Appraisal: Worth to Practice
Haroutounian, S., Ratz, Y., Ginosar, Y., Furmanov, K., Saifi, F, Meidan, R. & Davidson, E. (2016). The effect of medicinal cannabis on pain and quality-of-life outcomes in chronic pain. *Clinical Journal of Pain 32(12).* pp 1036-1043.	N/A	Open Label Study, single arm longitudinal study. (Cohort Study)	N=206

Ambulatory Pain Clinic in Jerusalem. | Pain reduction from baseline after 6 months using the S-TOPS.

Secondary: Baseline to 6 months Physical Disability, Family and Social Disability, Role-emotional disability, and Patient Satisfaction in relation to pain severity, pain interference and opioid consumption. | S-TOPS (Treatment Outcomes on Pain Survey-Short Form)

Brief Pain Inventory | Paired T-tests for normal distributed data. Linear regression analysis used to test the possible association between improved pain and deterioration in physical function. Significance set p<0.05 | Brief Pain Inventory scores improved from: 7.5 to 6.25 and pain interference score went from 8.14 to 6.71 post treatment p<0.001.

S-TOPS pain symptom scores and S-TOPS physical disability scale: 83.3 to 75. P<0.001.

Secondary Outcomes: All areas improved from baseline: p<0.001

32 of the 73 patients discontinued opioid treatment a 44% reduction. The medium opioid dose decreased from 60mg to 45mg however did not receive significance. | **Strengths:** 7-month study Significant number of parti cipants discontinued opioid treatment.

Low number of participants discontinued the study due to side effects: 11/206

Limitations: Smoked Cannabis No Control Group. Lack of periodic assessment of all adverse side effects. |

EFFECT OF CANNABIS ON PAIN AND QUALITY OF LIFE

Citation	Conceptual Framework	Design/Method	Sample/Setting	Major Variables Studied and Their Definitions	Measurement	Data Analysis	Findings	Appraisal: Worth to Practice
Narang, S., D., Gibson, A., Wasan, E., Ross, E., Michna, S. & Jamison, R. (2008). Efficacy of dronabinol as an adjuvant treatment for chronic pain patients on opioid therapy. *The Journal of Pain 5(3),* pp 254-264.	N/A	Phase I: Randomized single-dose double-blinded placebo-controlled crossover trial: participants received either 10mg or 20mg of dronabinol or placebo capsule (three 8-hour visits). Phase II: Extended open-label titrated trial of dronabinol as an addon medication to patients on stable doses of pioids.	Patients recruited from Brigham Women's Hospital and other affiliated teaching hospitals of Harvard Medical School. Phase I: n=30 Phase II: n=28	Examine the effect of cannabinoids on pain, improvements on sleep and mood.	Brief Pain Inventory Short form (BPI) a multi-dimensional pain questionnaire. (0-10 with 10 being the worst pain) Hospital Anxiety and Depression Scale (HADS) a 14 item self-report questionnaire which measures depression and generalized anxiety. Symptom Checklist, RAND 36- item Health Survey and the Medical Outcomes Study Sleep Scale (MOS)	SPSS Statistical Package for Social Sciences v13.0. Phase I used Fixed effects regression to assess longitudinal drug-related change in TOTPAR. Phase II: fixed effects regression modes to assess reported pain scores from baseline, changes in mood and antisfaction. Paired t tests were calculated for baseline versus end of study for: HADS, RAND-36, MOS.	Phase I: Total Pain Relief (TOTPAR) at 8 hours significantly greater in both 10mg and 20mg of dronabinol compared to placebo (20mg vs placebo p<.01) and (10mg drobinol vs placebo p<0.05). Average Pain Intensity: Drobinol vs. placebo u<.001) Phase II: Significant decrease in average pain scores from baseline p<.001. RAND significant improvement in Energy, Fatigue, Pain, and Social Functioning (p<.05, p<.01 and p<.01. MOS sleep scale showed decrease in sleep disturbance Phase I and Phase II <p.01. No significant difference in HADS score. No differences in pain relief between the 2 active treatment groups. Pain was reduced Sleep disturbances were significantly decreased and results suggest that dronabinol has a positive effect on sleep quality as well as pain.	Strengths: Robust Results Limitations: For my research, results did not measure any reduction in opioid use, patient were on stable doses of opioids. Long term use of cannabinoids was not addressed. Side effects such as dry mouth and lethargy were seen in the active treatment groups. Small Sample Size Some subjects had history of prior marijuana use. Placebo was not active.

EFFECT OF CANNABIS ON PAIN AND QUALITY OF LIFE

Citation	Conceptual Framework	Design/Method	Sample/Setting	Major Variables Studied and Their Definitions	Measurement	Data Analysis	Findings	Appraisal: Worth to Practice
Reiman, A., & Welty, M. & Solomon, P. (2017). Cannabis a a substitute for opiod-based pain medication: Patient self-report. *Cannabis and Cannabinoid Research 2*(1).	N/A	Cross Sectional Survey	2897 Medical Cannabis Patients. Pain was the most common condition for which respondents reported cannabis use (63%). N=841 reported using an opioid based pain medication over the past 6 months.	The use of cannabis as a substitute for opioid and nonopioid based pain medication.	Tilray Observational Patient Survey (TOPS)	Survey results. Patient Self Report.	97% of sample strongly agreed/agreed that they were able to decrease the amount of opioids they consume when they also use cannabis. 89% strongly agreed/agreed taking opioids produces unwanted side effects. 92% strongly agreed/agreed that cannabis has more tolerable side effects. 81% strongly agreed/agreed that cannabis was more effective in treating their condition than opioids. 71% strongly agreed/agreed that cannabis produces that same amount of pain relief than opioids.	**Strength:** Approved by the IRB at the University of California Berkeley. Supports published indicators that the permission of medical marijuana may decrease opioid related mortality, decrease spending on opioids and decrease traffic fatalities. **Limitations:** Survey Respondents were offered the chance to win a Firefly Vaporizer after participation in the survey. Patient self-report. No comparison groups. The title of the study was included in the invitation to participate which may have induced bias. Unable to determine how much cannabis participants used as well as strength variances.

22

EFFECT OF CANNABIS ON PAIN AND QUALITY OF LIFE

Citation	Conceptual Framework	Design/Method	Sample/Setting	Major Variables Studied and Their Definitions	Measurement	Data Analysis	Findings	Appraisal: Worth to Practice
Lynch, P. (2012). Cannabis as an adjunct to or substitute for opiates in the treatment of chronic pain. *Journal of Psychoactive Drugs, 44(2)*.	N/A	3 Single Subject Case Studies Patient 1: 47 year old multiple sclerosis person with headache, multisite joint pain, bladder spasm and leg spasticity. Patient 2: 35 year old HIV positive patient with painful peripheral neuropathy in lower limbs and hands. Patient 3: 44 year old patient with 6 year history of low back and left leg pain as a result of a work related fall.	3 Single Subject Case Studies	3 patients who used smoked marijuana in combination with an opioid. Patient 1: 2-4 puffs of marijuana at bedtime. Patient 2: 3-4 puffs 3-4 times daily. Patient 3: Several puffs to one joint 4-5 times daily.	Patient 1: 2-4 puffs of smoked marijuana at bedtime Patient 2: 3-4 puffs 3-4 times daily.	Patient 1: Pain, Opioid Use. Patient 2: Pain and Opioid Use. Patient 2: Pain and Opioid Use.	Patient 1: After six months of using marijuana, the patient's morphine was reduced from 75mg to 45mg daily, tizanidine from 24mg to 6mg once daily and Sertraline decreased from 150mg to 100mg daily. The patient reported improvement in pain, bladder spasms, spasticity and sleep. Patient 2: Prior to treatment patient using 300mg of long acting morphine daily and Gabapentin 2400 mg daily with continued pain of severe levels. After 4 months of treatment the patient's medication regime changed from: Morphine 180mg and after 9months the Morphine was discontinued along with the Gabapentin. Patient 3: Medication Regime prior to treatment Long Acting Morphine 150mg daily and Cyclobenzaprin 10mg three times daily. After treatment (2 weeks) he reduced Morphine to 90mg daily and after an additional two weeks to Morphine to 6omg daily and cyclobenzaprine to 10mg once daily.	**Strength:** These three real patients could reduce the use of Opioids by 60-100% when adding marijuana for pain management. **Limitation:** The source and strength of the medical marijuana is unknown. No standard measurements of pain were used.

23

EFFECT OF CANNABIS ON PAIN AND QUALITY OF LIFE

Citation	Conceptual Framework	Design/Method	Sample/Setting	Major Variables Studied and Their Definitions	Measurement	Data Analysis	Findings	Appraisal: Worth to Practice
							Patient reported that he could continue working and reported improved pain control.	

EFFECT OF CANNABIS ON PAIN AND QUALITY OF LIFE

Citation	Conceptual Framework	Design/Method	Sample/Setting	Major Variables Studied and Their Definitions	Measurement	Data Analysis	Findings	Appraisal: Worth to Practice
Johnson, J., Burnell-Nugent, M., Lossignol, D, Ganae-Motan, E, Potts, R. & Fallon, M. (2010). Multicenter, double-blind, randomized, placebo-controlled, parallel-group study of the efficacy, safety, and tolerability of thc:cbd extract and thc extract in patients with intractable cancer related pain. *Journal of Pain and Symptom Management* 39(2). Doi:10.1016/j.i painsymman.2 009.06.008	N/A	2-week multicenter, double-blind, randomized, placebo-controlled, parallel group trial.	N=177 patients with moderate to severe cancer related pain. THC-CBD (tetrahydrocannabinol) n=60 THC extract (n=58) Placebo (n=59) 3 centers in the United Kingdom	IV: THC-CBD THC placebo Extract DV=Pain, Quality of Life	Numerical Rating Scale (pain) Pain 0-10 Baseline rating. Visit 2 (7-10days) Visit 3 (14-20 days) rating The Brief Pain Inventory Short Form (BPI-SF). Quality of Life Questionnaire Version 3 (QLQ-C30) The European Organization for Research and Treatment of Cancer (EORTC) Adverse Events (AE)	Primary Analysis of Change (ANCOVA)	THC-CBD vs. Placebo - 1.37 vs. -0.67 statistically significant results on NRS. (Pain) p=0.014 THC vs. Placebo non-significant change in NRS -1.01 vs. -0.32 p=0.245 30% THC-CBD showed a reduction of more than 30% from baseline pain. No significant differences found in sleep quality, nausea scores. EORTC scores a worsening of nausea and vomiting with THC: CBD compared to placebo (P=0.02).	**Limitations:** Self-management of THC and THC: CBD. Limited to patients with intractable cancer related pain. **Strengths:** The study isolated one strand of Cannabinoid (THC: CBD) and compared it to THC and placebo.

25

EFFECT OF CANNABIS ON PAIN AND QUALITY OF LIFE

Citation	Conceptual Framework	Design/Method	Sample/Setting	Major Variables Studied and Their Definitions	Measurement	Data Analysis	Findings	Appraisal: Worth to Practice
Reynolds, D. & Osborn, H. (2013). The use of cannabinoids in chronic pain. *BMJ Case Report.* Doi: 10.1136/bcr-2013-010417.	N/A	Single Subject Case Study	N=1 Single Subject Case Study. Participant 56-year-old male with chronic pain following excision of facial cancer with poor analgesic control.	Management of Pain. Use of Nabilone 1mg twice daily.	Single Subject Reports.	Single Subject Report.	Patient reported pain control was greatly improved within days of starting Nabilone. Patient able to touch his face after not being able to do so after 4 years. Patient able to shave and got out in cold wet weather without pain and could hug loved ones again.	**Strength:** Real life applicability. **Limitations:** No control group. One subject report. Low sample size.

EFFECT OF CANNABIS ON PAIN AND QUALITY OF LIFE

Citation	Conceptual Framework	Design/Method	Sample/Setting	Major Variables Studied and Their Definitions	Measurement	Data Analysis	Findings	Appraisal: Worth to Practice
Vigil, J., Stith, S., Adams, I. & Reeves, A. (2017). Associations between medical cannabis and prescription opioid use in chronic pain patients: A preliminary cohort study. *PLOS ONE 12(11)*. DoI: 106084/m9figshare.5671721	N/A	Cohort Study: Preliminary and Historical Comparison to examine association between Medical Cannabis Program and Opioid Prescription Use	N=66 (Severe Chronic Pain Patients) Comparison Study no treatment or intervention. Medical Cannabis Program participant vs. comparison group opioid prescription participants Albuquerque, NM Rehabilitation Clinic	IV=Enrollment in the New Mexico Medical Cannabis Program DV=Pain Levels, Quality of Life, Social Life, Activity Levels, Concentration, and Opioid Usage Levels using longitudinal analysis	Changes in Pain Reduction Improved Quality of Life Survey Questionnaire Instrument measuring pain levels, effects of cannabis on quality of life, social life, activity levels and concentration. Patient records over a period of 21 months include refills of opioids Ceased opioid prescription Reduction in Opioid Usage	Logistic regression model to measure opioid use. Lease Square Approach to analyze the effect of the Medical Cannabis Program participation change n opioid use. Odds Ratio for dichotomous outcomes. Percentage change in prescriptions. Survey Results Confidence intervals: 95%.	Means Comparison on the Effect of Medical Cannabis Program Enrollment (MCP) on opioid prescription patterns. Ceased opioid prescriptions: p<0.001 Reduced opioid daily dosage p=0.001 Odds Ratio: (Baseline Odds 1.00 Survey: Pain Reduction in MCP participants (mean change 3.4) p<0.001 65% of participants reported great benefit to quality of life in MCP group. 52% reported great benefit to social life in MCP program. 47% of participants reported great benefit to activity levels and 41% reported greater benefit to levels of concentration.	**Limitations:** Single physician clinic participants. Small Sample Size Observational Nature Underpowered statistical analysis No medical supervision at the Medical Cannabis Program. Self-Managed Possible that patients received opioid treatment with multiple physicians **Strengths:** Study was approved by the Institutional Review Board at the University of New Mexico. MCP participants reported no adverse side effects of cannabis use. Study showed a strong correlation between enrollment in an MCP and cessation or reduction of opioid use.

EFFECT OF CANNABIS ON PAIN AND QUALITY OF LIFE

Citation	Conceptual Framework	Design/Method	Sample/Setting	Major Variables Studied and Their Definitions	Measurement	Data Analysis	Findings	Appraisal: Worth to Practice
Ware, M., Wang, T., Shapiro, S. & Collet, J. (2015). Cannabis for the management of pain: Assessment of safety study. Journal of Pain 16(12). Pp 1233-1242.	The safety of cannabis use by patients with chronic pain over one year.	Prospective Cohort Study with 1 year follow up.	N=431 7 clinics across Canada over 1 year. (6 and 12 months) Control Group:216 Cannabis Group: n=215	Primary Outcomes: Serious and Non- Serious Adverse Events Secondary Safety and Pulmonary and neurocognitive function and standard function and standard biochemistry, renal, hematology, liver, and endocrine function. Efficacy standards: Pain, mood, and quality of life.	Serious Adverse Events (SAE) Non- Serious Adverse Events. Adverse Events were measured using the World Health Organization Uppsala Monitoring Center Assessment System. Neurocognitive Function: 2 subtests using the Wechsler Memory Scale Pulmonary Function Test. Blood Test measured hematological, biochemical, liver, kidney, and endocrine function. Pain measured on visual analog scale using McGill Pain Questionnaire. Edmonton Symptom Assessment Scale, Profile Mood States. Quality of Life measured using the SF-36	Multiple Regression Analysis. Baseline vs. 6 months vs. 1 year	13% of C annabis group reported at least 1 SAE. 19% in control group reported SAE. Non- Serious Adverse Events: 88.4% of Cannabis group reported at least one non- serious adverse event and 85% of the control group reported at least one non- serious adverse event. Most common AE in cannabis group was nervous system (20%) and gastrointestinal (13.45%). Cannabis group had increased risk of non- serious adverse events Adjusted IRR=1.74 with 95% CI but not Serious Adverse Events. Increasing the daily dose of Cannabis did not lead to higher risks of SAE or AE. Neurocognitive: Significant Improvements in all subtest after 6 and 12 months. No differences were found between the control and intervention group after one year. Pulmonary Test: No change in vital capacity, functional residual capacity, and total lung	**Strengths:** First Cohort study of the long-term safety of medical cannabis ever conducted. **Findings:** Medical cannabis did not increase risks of serious adverse events but was associated with non-serious adverse events. Significant improvements in pain intensity and quality of life over 1 year among cannabis user's vs controls. **Limitations:** Small Sample Size and short follow up time. Significant drop out rate possible source of selection bias. Most cannabis group participants (66%) were experienced cannabis users. Not randomized controlled trial and allocation was not blinded.

28

EFFECT OF CANNABIS ON PAIN AND QUALITY OF LIFE

Citation	Conceptual Framework	Design/Method	Sample/Setting	Major Variables Studied and Their Definitions	Measurement	Data Analysis	Findings	Appraisal: Worth to Practice
							capacity over 1 year among the cannabis users. Blood Tests: No changes in liver, renal and endocrine function were observed. Pain: Compared to baseline a significant reduction in average pain intensity over 1 year was observed in the cannabis group: change −.92 CI−.63 1.23 and not in the control group. Quality of Life: Analysis of the change in PCS indicated greater improvement in physical function in cannabis users than in controls. 1.62 points after one year. Mood disturbance scale showed significant improvement for cannabis users compared with controls.	

29

YOUR KNOWLEDGE HAS VALUE

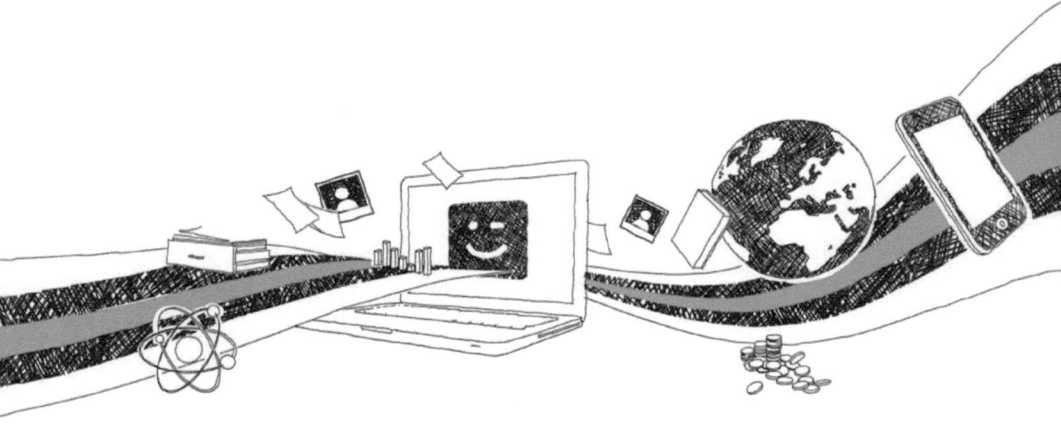

- We will publish your bachelor's and
  master's thesis, essays and papers

- Your own eBook and book -
  sold worldwide in all relevant shops

- Earn money with each sale

Upload your text at www.GRIN.com
and publish for free

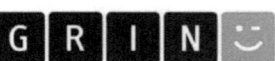